Closing the Deal

How to Pick Up Women

By Tommy Williams

Published by MuscleMag International
5775 McLaughlin Road
Mississauga, ON
Canada L5R 3P7

Designed by Jackie Thibeault

National Library of Canada Cataloguing in Publication

Williams, Tommy, 1962-
        Closing the deal : how to pick up women / by Tommy Williams.

ISBN 1-55210-032-4

        1. Dating (Social customs) 2. Man-woman relationships. I. Title.

HQ801.W54 2004   646.7'7'081   C2004-901145-6

Distributed in Canada by
CANBOOK Distribution Services
1220 Nicholson Road
Newmarket, ON
Canada L3Y 7V1

Distributed in the United States by
BookWorld Services
1941 Whitfield Park Loop
Sarasota, FL 34243

Printed in Canada

Table of Contents

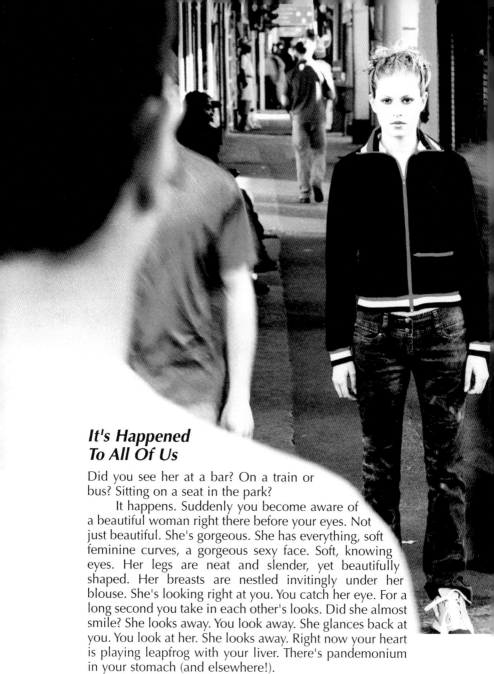

It's Happened
To All Of Us

Did you see her at a bar? On a train or
bus? Sitting on a seat in the park?

It happens. Suddenly you become aware of
a beautiful woman right there before your eyes. Not
just beautiful. She's gorgeous. She has everything, soft
feminine curves, a gorgeous sexy face. Soft, knowing
eyes. Her legs are neat and slender, yet beautifully
shaped. Her breasts are nestled invitingly under her
blouse. She's looking right at you. You catch her eye. For a
long second you take in each other's looks. Did she almost
smile? She looks away. You look away. She glances back at
you. You look at her. She looks away. Right now your heart
is playing leapfrog with your liver. There's pandemonium
in your stomach (and elsewhere!).

This is the woman for you. She's so sweet. What a
bed partner she would make! How can you possibly get to
know her? Perhaps she'll open the conversation? Not a

chance. What can you do? What will you do? Her thighs, my God, her thighs, they're moving. She gets up from her seat, a final glance your way and – she's gone. You watch her walk away. Out of your life. Her walk is elegant, yet sexy. Her behind caresses the inside of her dress with each delicious step. She's disappearing. Sashaying out of your life forever ...

You feel sorry for her because she doesn't know you. Yet in reality you are sorry for yourself because you don't know her. Angry at your cowardice, you tell yourself over and over again that you should have done something. You should have talked to her. She was beautiful, beautiful. And now she's gone.

You daydream about taking her out, about having fun, sharing jokes, places, people and things together. You dream about her being your woman. You tell yourself that you could have made her happy in bed. Yet there is less likelihood now, of you being the one to take her panties down tonight, than there is of Noah's Ark wending its way up the Mississippi. You, my friend have missed your chance. Another minor tragedy in your sex life.

It's not that you haven't had women. You have and what's more they've enjoyed you. You're pretty hot stuff with the ladies once you get to know them. But it's that initial getting to know them – the pick up – that isn't all that simple. Why? Because you don't like the idea of rejection. You don't like the idea of being ignored, or even worse, her telling you to get lost. Or reporting you to the nearest cop. Or both!

In the days and weeks to come you think of her. The exact appearance of her face may have dimmed a little in your memory. But you do remember that she was utterly sensational. The tastiest female you've ever seen. Why didn't you make contact with her? There must have been a way to have gotten to know her. Some magic technique that would have made her come with you. Talk to you. Like you, and eventually sleep with you.

Well, the fact is, there is a way. In truth there are thousands of ways. Too bad you didn't apply one to that woman but at least after you have read this book you will know what to do next time.

It's Only Natural

Being introduced to a woman in your home (by your aunt?) or at a party (by your cousin?) is an easy way to start up an acquaintance. A relationship can develop, almost naturally. Because, well it's all been set up for you. But as luck would have it, your aunt or cousin don't seem to introduce you to the type of women that you are looking for.

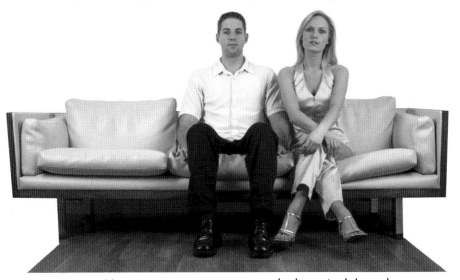

No, you want more; you want the best. And the only way you're going to get these real beauties is by working on your own.

Basically the secret behind 'pulling birds' as the English would say, is chat. Talk. You have to get a two-way conversation going. The nice thing about this essential chat, is that it doesn't matter one bit what you actually say, as long as it's mainly nonsense. Don't come on too heavy with new women. It can scare them off. Traditional pickup lines, however, are a no-no.

Let me explain:

When you see an attractive woman on a bus, in a restaurant, at a museum, in a line-up or on the subway, a woman that you desperately want to go out with, and take to bed, you fail to make an approach because you have a fear of rejection. You can't bear the thought of her turning you down. This is lesson number one – building self-confidence. It is essential. Learn not to be afraid.

Don't come on too heavy. It can scare women off.

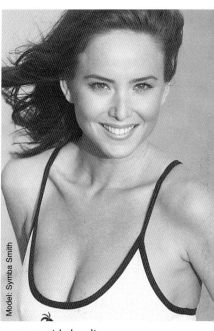

Model: Symba Smith

Have you ever noticed that some of the fellows that regularly go out with the most beautiful-looking women, are actually themselves, less than good looking. In fact, many are downright plain. I myself, and I hate to admit it, am spectacularly ordinary. Certainly nearer the ugly end of the scale, rather than the good looking side. I'm not rich, well-built, even remotely striking, yet being unimpressive as I am, hasn't kept me from falling head over heels in love with outstanding women. I'm crazy about them. My whole life is built around that most delicious word – seduction!

I've got a lot of catching up to do because I only mastered the secret to picking up women recently. Up until that time I was content with leading an ordinary life with very ordinary dull women. True I had my fun, but life was never like this. Now, I'm on top of the world – gleefully happy. Believe me, if an ordinary guy like me can learn to pick up women, you can become an expert.

Fear Can Paralyze A Man

It's rather sad really. On the one hand you have thousands of sexy looking women dressed up to the hilt, tight jeans, high firm breasts, long elegant thighs, and so on; yet most guys are afraid to try to pick them up because they do not

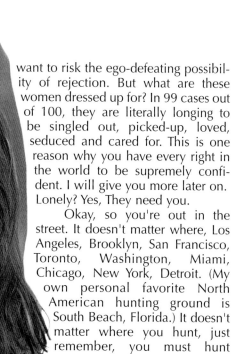

want to risk the ego-defeating possibility of rejection. But what are these women dressed up for? In 99 cases out of 100, they are literally longing to be singled out, picked-up, loved, seduced and cared for. This is one reason why you have every right in the world to be supremely confident. I will give you more later on. Lonely? Yes, They need you.

Okay, so you're out in the street. It doesn't matter where, Los Angeles, Brooklyn, San Francisco, Toronto, Washington, Miami, Chicago, New York, Detroit. (My own personal favorite North American hunting ground is South Beach, Florida.) It doesn't matter where you hunt, just remember, you must hunt alone. Don't take a friend.

Men are afraid to approach beautiful women for fear of rejection.

Women do not respond so readily to the advances of two or more guys. Keep to the one-on-one strategy and you'll enjoy a higher rate of success.

Remember women get lonely, very lonely. Hard to believe maybe, but it's true.

This is a little chauvinistic of me, but still true for the greater part: women rely on good, strong heterosexual relationships to keep them happy and contented. And if they're not in the

Model: Angie Chittenden

Don't take a friend. Women do not respond so readily to the advances of two or more guys.

middle of one – they are lonely. The next time you see a beautiful woman strolling down the street, bear my words in mind. Both men and women tend to settle into a relationship that is not what they really want. They are still looking.

She's done-up-to-the-hilt for a reason. Her ass looks sexy, high, firm and inviting for a reason. She didn't just ask the shopkeeper for any pair of jeans. She probably tried as many as a dozen pairs on to get the right effect. Why? Because she wanted to look sexy, attractive, inviting. Who for? Her mother, sister, boyfriend? Maybe, but unlikely (especially if she's out in the street or at a bar). No, chances are she's doing it for you. She may not admit it, even to herself.

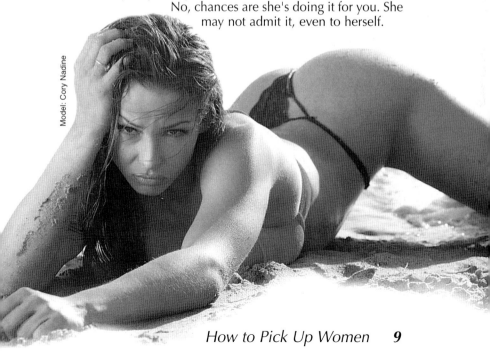

Model: Cory Nadine

Few women will openly admit that they want to be "picked up" but never the less it is a categorical fact, that done in the correct way, an attractive woman can be picked up in the street with unbelievable ease. Not

Women are just as sex oriented as guys.

because of any particular skill of the men who try, but because inherently, they want to be picked up. It's what life is all about. It's natural. Women rely on it today more

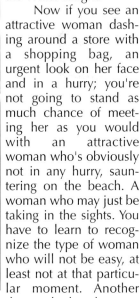

than at any other time. They are still looking for the White Knight.

Now if you see an attractive woman dashing around a store with a shopping bag, an urgent look on her face and in a hurry; you're not going to stand as much chance of meeting her as you would with an attractive woman who's obviously not in any hurry, sauntering on the beach. A woman who may just be taking in the sights. You have to learn to recognize the type of woman who will not be easy, at least not at that particular moment. Another day, she could be less harassed, less rushed and consequently more receptive to being approached.

Know Your Prey

Think of it this way. If a woman told you that you had very attractive legs or a sensual back, it would make you pretty receptive towards her right? You bet it would. Well, women are just as sex orientated as us guys. Tell them how much

10   *Closing the Deal*

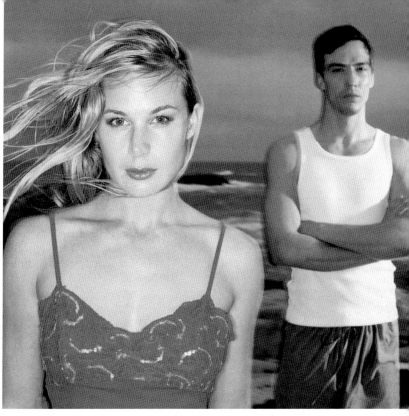

you appreciate them and they'll turn on to you! Why do you think women parade around in clothes that emphasize their sexual parts? Why have so many of them stopped wearing bras and panties? Just to look pretty? Yes! But mainly to look beddable! To make you want to go to bed with them. To make you long to caress and fondle their bodies and to ultimately enjoy the ecstasy of meaningful sexual intercourse.

Get Serious

The fact that you are reading this book indicates that you are serious about bedding luscious women. But make sure that you do mean business. For nothing is worse than a half-hearted pick-up.

A woman will sense that you are serious and it will turn her on.

Every, even halfway experienced woman, has suffered abuse and hurt at the hands of some fellow or another. They don't like to be made a fool of. Take it from me; when you pick up a woman you have to show her that you mean business. A woman will sense that you are serious and it will turn her on. If she thinks that you are just chatting her up to show off to your pals, or just for a 5-minute gig; she'll back off.

Before she makes any kind of commitment to you she wants to be certain that you're going to take her up on it.

Nothing enrages an attractive woman more than a once attentive man who makes a pass and then backs off at the last moment. It makes her feel rejected and foolish!

One of the best picker-uppers I know is Richard. He works around New York, Greenwich Village in the Big Apple.

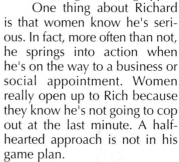

One thing about Richard is that women know he's serious. In fact, more often than not, he springs into action when he's on the way to a business or social appointment. Women really open up to Rich because they know he's not going to cop out at the last minute. A half-hearted approach is not in his game plan.

Only positive action gets results.

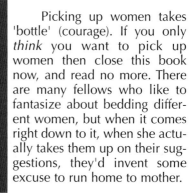

Picking up women takes 'bottle' (courage). If you only *think* you want to pick up women then close this book now, and read no more. There are many fellows who like to fantasize about bedding different women, but when it comes right down to it, when she actually takes them up on their suggestions, they'd invent some excuse to run home to mother.

So be sure that you want to go through with it. Don't be a dreamer. The very fact that you're serious is more important than the possessing of devastating good looks or great charm and wit!

Wishing is only wishing. It means nothing. Only positive action gets results.

Appearance

As I suggested to you, I have a face like the back of a bus! It used to bother me, but no more. Don't let the lack of good looks dampen your spirit, or sap your confidence. Studies have shown conclusively, that experienced women are not so superficial as men. In other words, they are more interested in what a man has inside than what he looks like. On the other hand there are literally hundreds of thousands of men who would choose as a partner, a woman who had an amazing bod over a more intelligent or genuine woman whose body was less than perfect. But

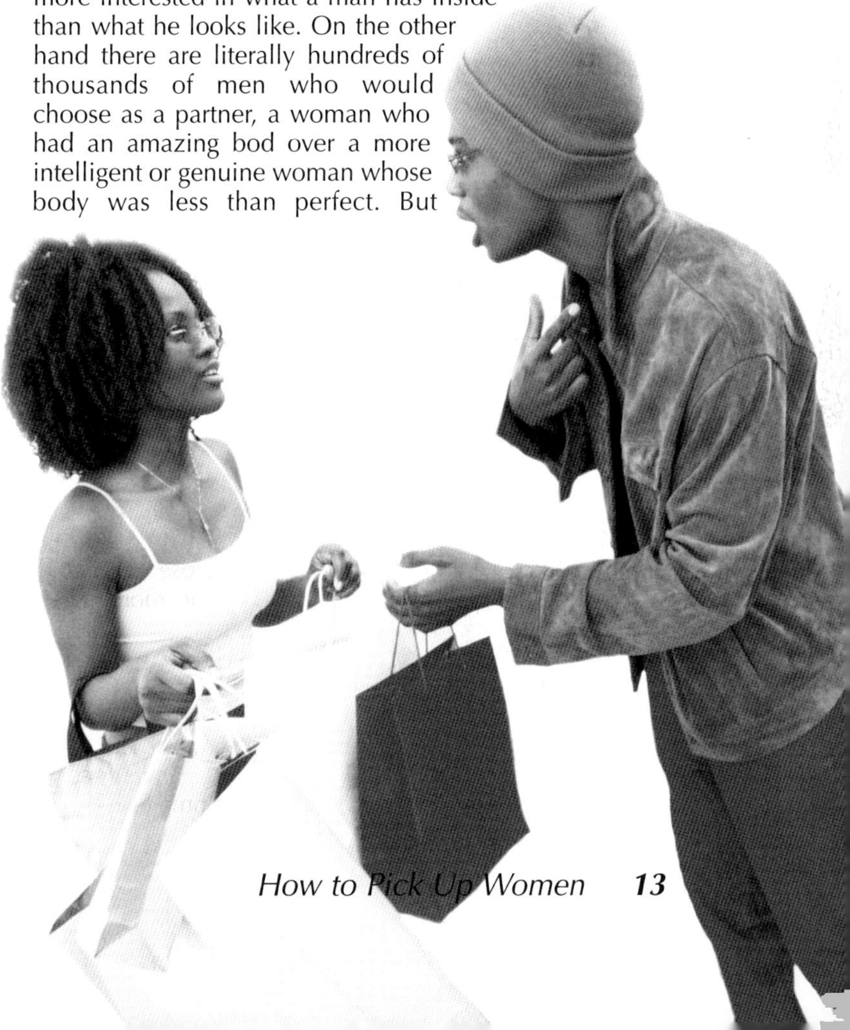

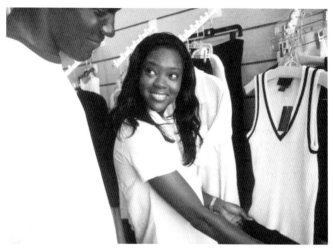

women, bless 'em, are different. They go for what is said to them rather than what their eyes see. "It's the warmth and attentiveness of a man that turns me on," said one attractive blonde I was talking to recently, "I couldn't care less about his looks."

Warning: Whereas women generally don't regard good looks as important, it should be noted that basic fundamentals like hygiene, clean clothes and decent manners should be regarded as assets towards the ultimate 'pulling' power of a man.

Many women have told me that they actually prefer men who are not very good looking.

"They have better personalities, are more interesting, and they don't just lie back and rely on their looks. A man who is not a natural Adonis has to compensate by improving his flare, talk and personality. I look for warmth in a man. If he is not warm, and interesting, his looks are not worth a damn and if he is warm and interesting, I don't give a damn what he looks like."

Don't let the lack of good looks dampen your spirit, or sap your confidence.

Many women claim that they react to a person, not his looks. Women are seduced by men who approach them in a nice way. Men who can talk; men who are interesting and warm. Looks are at the bottom of the list. This is often hard for men to understand because to many men a woman's looks are of utmost importance. Any woman who doesn't have a pretty face and a bathing beauty's body is at once discarded from their minds.

But women are different. They are turned on by what we are and not what we appear to be, and we should thank them for it!

Using Props and Circumstances

Some years ago in England a friend of mind named Zol (that's his real name, he was Hungarian) used to amaze me with his ability to pick up women. But he was only able to do it if he had an excuse. He wasn't daring enough to go up to a woman *cold turkey* and give her a line. But heaven help any woman who was overloaded with shopping bags, carrying or walking a dog, trying to hail a cab, or a woman trying on clothes in a store. Zol could turn any of these circumstances into masterpieces of picking-up artistry. "You've got enough food there for both of us," he would say to the lady with a bulging basket of groceries, and with a hungry look on his face. If he got a smile, he would continue. "I haven't had a square meal in weeks."

More often than not of course, these women were on their way home to a husband or boyfriend, but Zol hadn't actually risked being rejected because he hadn't requested anything and had not been turned down. He got a high failure rate with his play-safe lines, but then he never felt rejected, which was important to him. And naturally, if his early remarks were

Women are seduced by men who approach them in a nice way.

received warmly he would pursue the woman and yes, sometimes even get asked home for a meal (and more). It so happened that he was a good cook, and he often persuaded the woman by asking, "How do you make your gravy? Listen, I can show you how to make a gravy that will make the taste buds in your mouth cry out for more."

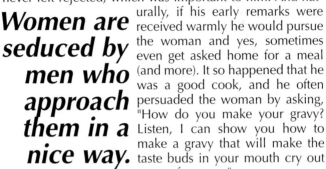

To a woman trying clothes on in a store, he would say: "That color compliments your complexion. You look terrific!" or "Its been a long time since I've seen a coat worn so elegantly. You look fabulous!" or "If I was a millionaire I would buy that dress for you. It's great!" "Say, what kind of a dog is that?" he would ask a lady dog owner. "He's kind of cute" or "Do you want to sell that dog? He's the sweetest little fella I've ever seen." Crafty Zol knew only too well that women love their pets, and were always melted by compliments about their little doggies.

Using circumstances and props whenever possible will aid your picking up ability. Why? Because it adds authenticity to the whole getting-to-know-you business. The greatest (and most unlikely) circumstances I ever had to aid me in making a pickup, was when a political bomb went off outside the *Hard Rock* restaurant in London, England years ago. I was in the restaurant at the time try-

Keep your eyes open for props and circumstances to help you.

ing to think of a line I could use to get to know some attractive American girls sitting nearby. And I tell you, when that bomb went off we all became very good friends in a matter of minutes. In fact, we all went from the Hard Rock to a little club I know, and from there...

Keep your eyes open for props and circumstances to help you. You will be surprised at how many different circumstances there are, and the extraordinary way in which they can help you get women to respond more readily.

Cold Turkey Pickup

Many consider that picking a woman up in the street, with no aid of props and circumstance, to be the hardest of all. This of course depends on numerous conditions. Personally, if I see a woman rushing down the road, almost running, I would not dream of trying to pick her up. She's obviously got other priorities. Let her be. Look out for the unrushed, unattached woman. The one who is window shopping, the casual walker, the stroller. This is where you are likely to score.

Here she comes – sashaying towards you. A moderate walk, a slightly

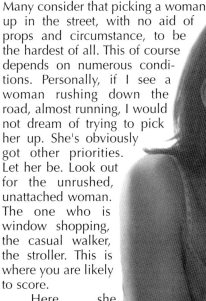

aloof look on her face. Your heart is starting to speed up. Uh! Uh! What do we do? What do we say? Quick, check her out. Anything special about her? Try and learn in a few seconds what type she is: Sophisticated? A dancer? Intellectual? A secretary, an actress, stewardess, a waitress? Is there anything about her you could remark on? What to do?

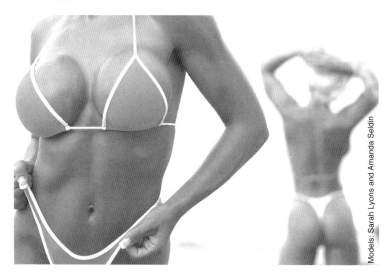

Models: Sarah Lyons and Amanda Seldin

The answer to that is – almost anything. As long as you keep talking, why not try?

"Excuse me, I just had to tell you that you're the nicest looking woman I've ever seen. Come and have a coffee. There's a place just across the road."

OR

(Smile) "Didn't I meet you in the lounge at the Istanbul Hilton?" (This is a good one. She may be impressed that you're a world traveller and flattered that you think she's one, too.)

OR

"When I see someone like you I thank my lucky stars I'm not married."

OR

"Who the heck is your dentist? You have the greatest looking teeth."

18   *Closing the Deal*

1. "Who the heck is your hairdresser? You have the most beautiful hair."

2. "Who the heck is your agent? You're one of the greatest looking models I've ever seen."

3. "Who the heck is your manicurist? Your hands are exquisite."

4. "Where do you buy your clothes? They look fabulous."

OR

"You're Aquarius, aren't you?" (Whether she is or not, she'll be interested. Most girls are fascinated by astrology.) And once in a while you'll even guess correctly. And that should lead to some real curiosity and intrigue about how on earth you should know a thing like that.

Sometimes you may find yourself sitting near a woman in a bar, in a plane, a restaurant or even in a line-up and there is no need to deliver a specially concocted or extravagant line. Under such circumstances you can

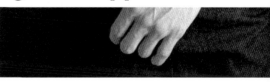

Be ready for those golden opportunities.

simply remark on the weather, or the terrible coffee, cold food or marvellous view or ask the time. From then on easy communication can flow and you don't have to endure the strain of high pressure or clever conversation.

Lucky Breaks

Once in a while, a golden opportunity comes your way. And man you should be ready for it. Success is opportunity meeting preparedness. I suppose that I've had about thirty lucky breaks in my life, and regrettably I have only taken advantage of the last two. The other twenty-eight times I was just too chicken or inexperienced to act. I lost out! And I regret it to this day.

In my time I have found myself sitting next to a real beauty of a woman on a transatlantic plane (didn't even manage to utter a 'hello' or a 'goodbye'). I have been next to a young well-known model when she slipped on a wet San Francisco pavement and was unable to get up. (I was so slow to the rescue that an old lady actually helped her up and did the comforting.) I have been in a stuck elevator with a sex bomb and couldn't turn the situation into any

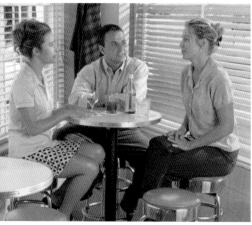

type of relationship. I have carried an attractive girl from a crashed car and not had the guts to even call her at the hospital to find out how she was coming along. Golden opportunities I have had, and golden opportunities I have blown.

Should you have a lucky break, a golden opportunity then be prepared for it. It is madness not to take advantage of lucky breaks that throw you and a terrific woman together. True, they don't happen that often. All the more reason for you to jump into action when these occasions present themselves. Never has the boy scouts credo "Be prepared" been more relevant.

Success is opportunity meeting preparedness.

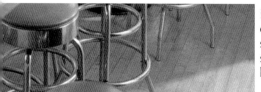

What Turns A Woman On?

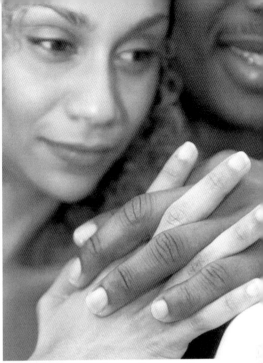

There's really no way of figuring it out. Women can be turned on by a thousand and one things; little things.

We men are not half as creative in the things we like about the opposite sex. In fact, ninety percent of us are either 'bottom men' or 'breast men'. We all like facial good looks and that's about it. A few schmo's are into feet – c'est la vie.

Take advantage of lucky breaks that throw you together with a terrific woman.

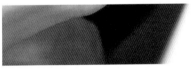

But women are different. They can be turned on by the appearance of a man's fingernails! One woman I know confided that she fell in love with her husband because of the hair on his wrists. She explained with rapture how "the dark hairs fell lovingly across his square wrist bones ..." Actually, I couldn't see much difference between his wrists and the next mans but it was certainly obvious enough to her. I knew her husband before they were married and he had been breaking his neck for years to be a success with women. If only he had known that all he had to do was roll up his sleeves!

Many women, it seems are turned on by hands, especially medium to large hands. If you possess pretty rugged (and clean) hands then lose no time putting 'palms together' with likely candidates. You may just score a gigantic success. In his famous book *How to Pick Up Girls* author Eric Weber describes how one woman gave herself totally to a man because of his cute feet!

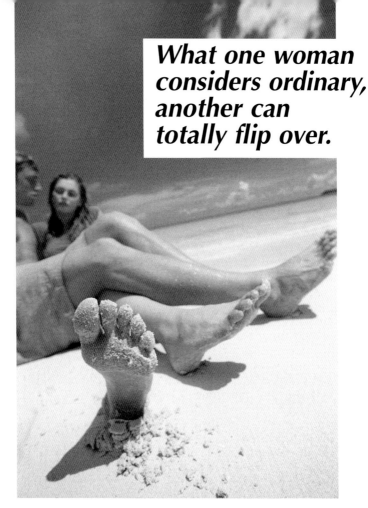

What one woman considers ordinary, another can totally flip over.

In the video *Six Women* (mail-order orderline 1-888-254-0767), fitness women declared that in their opinion the sexiest part of a man was his forearms.

You may not consider yourself to be the most handsome fellow around, but you can be sure that there are plenty of things about you that girls will love. It may be something that you hadn't even considered – your eyes, feet, nose (big noses are often a favorite), hands, hips, back, cheekbones, teeth, smiles, hair (both hirsute and baldies have their appeal), skin, the clothes you wear, or even your eyelashes. Many women rely on a quick glance at a man's shoes to decide on whether or not he is worth even talking to. All can be a turn on. And the remarkable thing is that what one woman considers ordinary, another

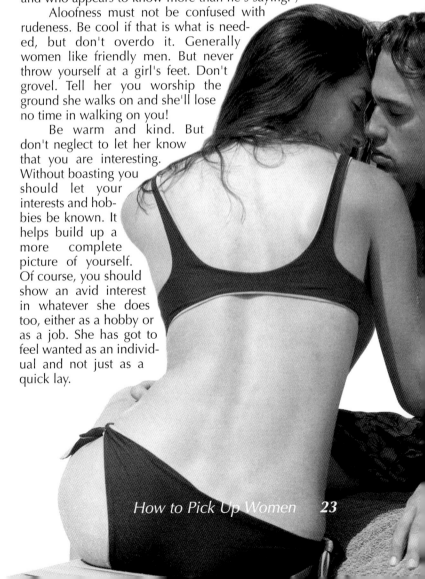

can totally flip over. I'll never forget one womans reaction to a short, overweight bald man who asked her to a dance. "He's so dumpy and cuddly," she squirmed, "I hope he asks me to go home with him!"

One important thing that turns women on to men is their attitude. A sexy girl told me that she could tell if a complete stranger on the other side of the room was attractive or desirable (even if he wasn't good looking) by his facial expression. ("I like a man who is moderately aloof and who appears to know more than he's saying.")

Aloofness must not be confused with rudeness. Be cool if that is what is needed, but don't overdo it. Generally women like friendly men. But never throw yourself at a girl's feet. Don't grovel. Tell her you worship the ground she walks on and she'll lose no time in walking on you!

Be warm and kind. But don't neglect to let her know that you are interesting. Without boasting you should let your interests and hobbies be known. It helps build up a more complete picture of yourself. Of course, you should show an avid interest in whatever she does too, either as a hobby or as a job. She has got to feel wanted as an individual and not just as a quick lay.

Don't Be a Meany!

One of the greatest turn-offs for women is to be approached by an aggressive guy. Gone are the days (if they ever existed) of the typical rough 'n' tough Bob Mitchum or Humphrey Bogart movie styles...

You'd be surprised how many guys actually use nastiness as a basis for attempting a pickup.

"Bogey" may have been loved and adored on the screen but he wouldn't have lasted long with his ornery, mean behavior in reality away from the fantasy of his celluloid image.

Women go for the nice, warm, friendly types. Approach a woman in a bar and tell her that she's a little old to be going braless and she'll hate you. Common sense? Yes, but you'd be surprised at how many guys actually use nastiness as a basis for attempting a pickup. Actually, it's a kind of a buffer to their ego. If a guy starts off a conversation with a woman by being rude or aggressive, then he has nothing to lose if she turns him down. He can always claim that he wasn't trying to pick up the dumb chick anyway. "Just trying to get a rise out of her."

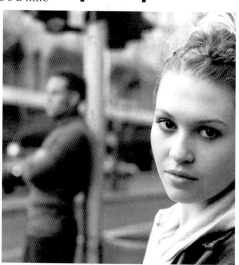

Remember that when you are approaching a woman for the first time, you have to make a pretty favorable impression. You have to come across as a warm, sincere, friendly type of fellow, who's enchanted enough with a girl to want to meet her.

She doesn't know you from Adam. In fact, she's got to make up her mind pretty quickly whether she's going to be nice to you or tell you to get lost. Give her 'agro' and

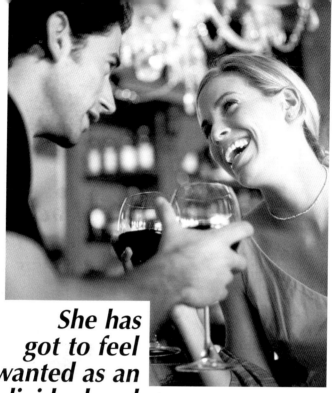

She has got to feel wanted as an individual and not just as a quick lay.

she'll knock you and your ego into next week with a resounding rejection that you may not easily forget.

Bear in mind that it is difficult for a woman to be hurtful to someone who shows her kindness and warmth. It's your best investment.

Be Complimentary

Women thrive on compliments. Even when they know you are lying through your teeth. They enjoy the luxury of being paid the eternal compliment, especially if you are clever enough to point out something rather obscure that they may have overlooked or at most, not given much thought to.

"You have the sweetest earlobes" may go down well or, "It's been a long time since I've seen such pretty feet" How about? "I love the way your nails grow." Or, "What sensational eyes you have, I can't take my eyes off them!" Or, "That's the most flawless looking nose I've seen in years!"

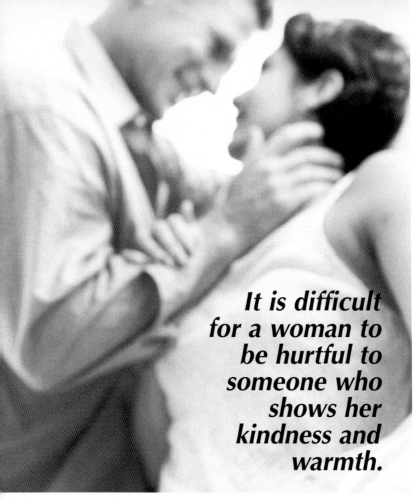

It is difficult for a woman to be hurtful to someone who shows her kindness and warmth.

Be aware of complimenting unless there is at least some foundation for your praise. You'll wreck everything if you tell her that her fingernails are gorgeous when in fact they are chewed up to her knucklebones. Likewise, it is pointless making a thing of earlobes if in fact she has the kind of ears that have no lobes (yes, they exist!). Also, stay clear of complimenting her on any obvious sexual quali- ties she may possess. "You have luscious big tits," will not usually impress so much as: "Your shoulders are really beautifully shaped." Your more personal remarks can come later. They will be enjoyed more once you get to know her, but for pick-up reasons it is usually (though not always) more desirable to keep your compliments on a higher, more sophisticated plain. The important point is to visual- ly search for something about her that is in fact remarkable, and you will score more brownie points if you compliment something that she is hardly aware of.

Women spend a lot of time in making themselves look attractive. They go through a thousand moods where they fluctuate from happiness to despondency, all over the way they look. They can vary from being completely confident over what they look like, to being utterly depressed. It may not make sense to us men, but it is true. Accordingly, your compliment can mean more than you'll ever know. Flattery, especially when it is truly delivered and honestly felt, can get you everywhere with a woman. Don't water your comments down. Lay them on thick. She will love you for it – literally.

Don't Put On An Act

In a sense, you're going to have to put on an act when you approach a woman for the first time. But don't make the mistake of coming across like a professional. Learn to relax. Don't talk too quickly. Say what you have to say in a kind, warm sort-of-way. Try and smile.

Flattery, especially when it is truly delivered and honestly felt, can get you everywhere.

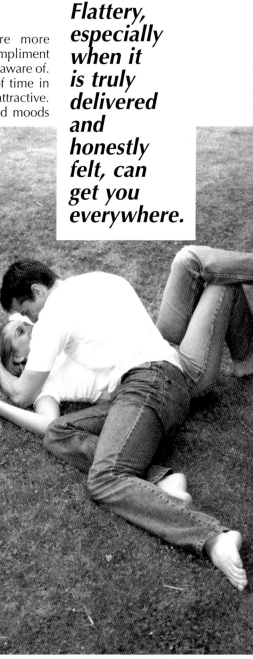

Remember that the worst thing that can happen to you is that she'll ignore you. So what?

You're not going to be worried by that. She may even tell you to leave her alone. Okay, so you do. No great shakes. You'll still survive. It's not a matter of life and death. Actually, as I've said before, if you approach a woman with a smile and a warm friendly attitude, you're going to get very little 'agro' anyway. Your worst moments may never culminate from anything more direct than: "Thank you for your offer, but I'm happily married." Why, she may even like you, but because of certain circumstances, simply has to turn you down. The point is, there is no reason for despondency or to feel rejected. It happens to us all from time to time. Your successful conquests will far outnumber outright rejections. Remember, the most famous and important people in the world suffer defeat of some kind during their lives, time and time again. Without wishing to seem harsh it should be pointed out that getting your feelings hurt is part of life. Don't be over sensitive.

When attempting to pick up a woman, try and be yourself. Women often get a sixth sense about a guy if he seems too practiced or fluent. On the other hand, if you only manage to garble out a few animal noises, you're not going to make much of an impression anyway.

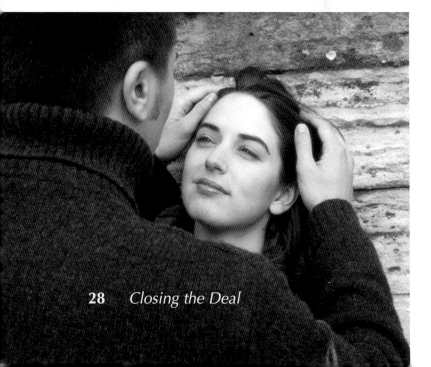

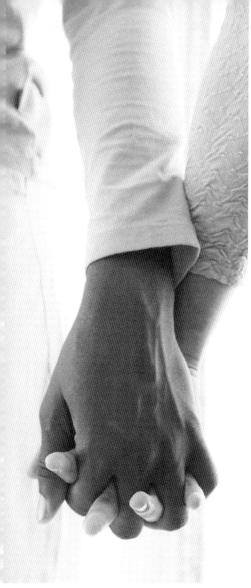

But I'll tell you something, the majority of women would rather be approached by a fellow who was a little shy and not that smooth, than by a flippant know-it-all who delivered line-after-line of practiced verbiage. A man who is too aggressive can frighten off a woman. She could get the feeing that the guy picks up women for a living. Scores of them day-after-day-after-day.

Now this may well become the case. But you must not allow your picking up to become too slick. Each woman you meet must be made to feel that she is the only woman in the world for you. She must feel that you are utterly enchanted with not just her outward appearance but her very essence and inward personality. Women would like to believe that you were just strolling by and suddenly noticed them, not just as an attractively shaped piece of physical femininity, but as a complete woman, full of the excitement and mystery of Napoleon's Josephine or Mark Anthony's Cleopatra.

Hence the unusual success of the following lines:

A man who is too aggresssive can frighten off a woman.

"I've never done this before but there is something different about your eyes that makes me want to know you."
OR

"You have an inward quality that I can't put my finger on. I just had to say hello."
OR

"Hey, listen, something about you just makes my knees weak. For the life of me, I can't tell you what it is but I just had to speak to you."

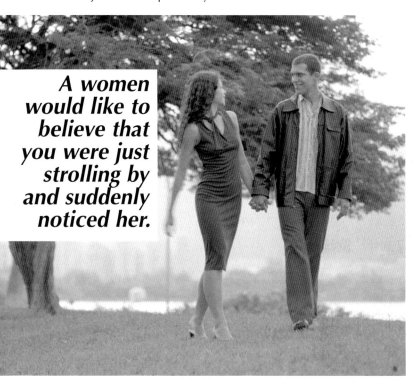

A women would like to believe that you were just strolling by and suddenly noticed her.

Straight Forward Often Does It!

I delivered some pretty extraordinary lines to some women. Some lines have raised a laugh; others have raised an eyebrow. My verbal masterpieces have often pleased me and yet died when it came to their 'pulling' ability.

I think it is often not what one says, but rather, how one says it, that is important. Even the old oddball corny lines of yesteryear can work wonders if delivered with the right panache.

"What's a nice girl like you doing in a place like this?"

"What's a nice girl like you doing in a place like this?"

Or, "Don't I know you from somewhere?" are prime examples of overworked lines, yet both can still work wonders if delivered with sincerity. You see, it's how you say it! Although certain girls really dig a guy who says something original and unique, there are many times when the most straight forward and direct approach is best.

One woman confided to me that she prefers a man who simply asks the time or remarks casually on the weather. "Forget the false charm and phoney wit and give me a fellow who simply says, "Hello." Another told me. "I don't like to be shot a line. I really go for a guy who comes up to me at a party, or something, and says: "You look interesting, what's your name?" Or, "I couldn't help but notice you from across the room – you look nice." Any man who is straight forward like this, gets my full attention. I love him for it, and admire him for his direct approach.

A friend of mine in Texas has just one line. He enjoyed about a twenty percent success rate using it – "Listen" he says, "I know this sounds silly, but I'm fairly sure I've fallen in love with you."

Now this line borders between *direct* and the *preposterous*. Accordingly, it works well with some

Some lines work well with some women and bomb badly with others.

women yet bombs badly with others. Also, he found it worked best with women whom he had only just seen. If he delivered it after knowing a girl for a few hours, then he was liable to get a smirk rather than a smile. Curious facts, but certainly true in the case of my Texas friend.

There is a happy knack that you can acquire, of seeming to be straight forward with a woman, yet in reality you'll be lying through your teeth.

"Didn't you go to Cincinnati Art School?" is a 'beaut, because 99 out of 100 girls will sincerely believe that you are genuine in wanting to know. Incidentally, it may be a good idea for you to have actually attended Cincinnati Art School since these lines, if delivered often enough have a funny way of getting one into hot water. I mean if you've never even been to Cincinnati what do you do if the girl replies "No, but my father has been the principal there for the last 14 years!"

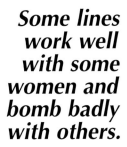

Model: Christina Bybee

The vast majority of women picked up will not end up in bed with the man.

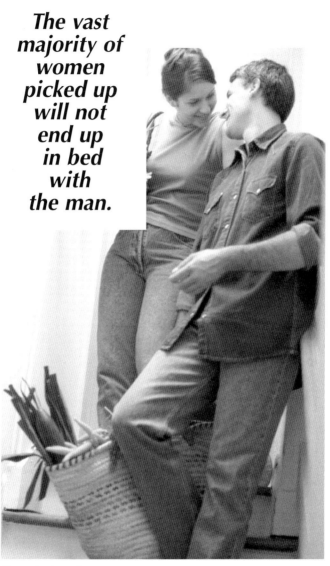

Don't Rush Her

One guy I knew just had to have a different woman each night of the week. It was an education watching him work at it. At 10:30 p.m. he was very choosey about what girls he would try and chat up. At 11:30 he was not so choosey and would condescend to talk to less attractive girls. At

12:30 he would take anything! His lifelong ambition was to rush a woman, usually any woman, to bed. That was his 'thing'. Now, most red-blooded men want to get at least their fair share of bedroom gymnastics, but I feel that the importance of taking a woman to bed the moment you meet her is overstated. There are many women who are just not cut out for rushing into bed with a man before they even know his name. There has to be friendship, a degree

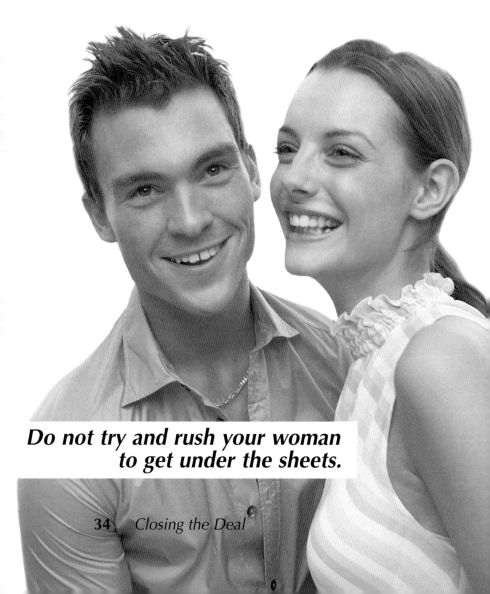

Do not try and rush your woman to get under the sheets.

of fondness and meaningfulness for most women. True, there are women who will be as keen to get into your pants as you are to get into their panties, but this is not true in most cases.

As you know, men are always bragging about their latest conquests. Many tell stories of laying women that just are not true. The fact is that the vast majority of women picked up will not end up in bed with the man, at least not the first night. And why should they? But, from the stories you hear from other men you would think they pick up women, every so often and 'lay' each and every one of them within minutes.

It is advisable that you not try and rush to get your women under the sheets. Give it time. A date or two, a movie, a few drinks and both of you will probably enjoy the sexual side more, because of the development of genuine regard for each other, over a period of several days; perhaps even weeks. Doubtless, there will be quick 'screws' in your life. It would be a crime to leave a wanton girl in a state of want, if she had clearly shown that she was as horny as all hell, and in need of relief.

My advice is that you take your time and not rush your newly picked maidens. Most will like you for your patience, and your reticent action may even prompt them to make the initial sexual advances, which in itself makes a pleasant uplifting change. N'est pas?

Where To Meet Women

The question of where to meet women has bothered some people enormously. It all depends, of course on what you're looking for. If you think the women in your neighborhood are terrific then you need look no further. You can develop your 'home ground'. On the other hand, if you

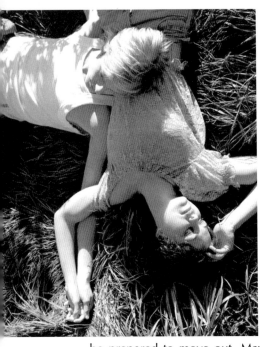

really like a variety of extraordinary women, then you may have to move to the big city. (Generally speaking the bigger cities have the most attractive looking females.)

Don't get me wrong, you can spend the rest of your life right where you are, and have enormous success. The point I am making is that if your lust is such that you do not have a wide enough choice where you are at present then you should be prepared to move out. Maybe you'll only want to be away from home one day a week. On the other hand you may want to try and find a job in the big city and enjoy happy hunting for a number of years.

The wonderful thing about large cities (like New York or Los Angeles) is that they have just about any type of woman you could possibly desire to meet. Even the thought of it can be quite breathtaking (gasp!).

Most big North American cities have different areas, which lend themselves to specific types of women. The first thing you have to do is work out just what type of woman it is that you would like to meet. After you decide then some research is necessary. A lot of super women can be found in muse-

Half your battle may be in finding the women.

ums, art galleries, zoos, swimming areas, skating rinks, libraries, restaurants, hotel lobbies, parks, train stations as well as the more obvious places like singles bars, coffee bars, drinking halls, dance establishments. Often, it can be a good idea, when visiting a new city, to find out where the big shopping centers are. Most women seem to shop at boutiques as opposed to the large, cheap chain stores. Half your battle may be in finding the women. The other half in finding the words. Whatever the case, you're going to succeed. That I am sure of!

Cameras

A friend of mine is almost never without a camera around his neck. The sole purpose of his taking up photography is to aid his pickup chances. And it's not such a bad idea, if you are a shy type.

My friend reasons that there are a few attractive women in the world who are not intrigued over having their picture taken. He's gone to the trouble of having business cards printed which read: "Simon James, photographer" plus his address and telephone number. Thus, his authenticity as a photographer is further demonstrated. He

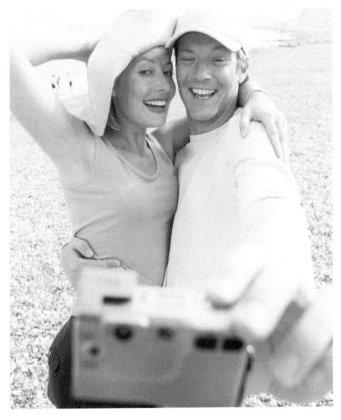

Photography can aid a man who feels he needs a real excuse for approaching women.

gives these cards out anywhere he can at about the rate of ten a day. He gets results too. Actually his pictures are nothing special, but the women he meets in this way are!

The good thing about photography is that:

a. It gives you an excuse to stop the woman in the first place. i.e. "Excuse me, you are extremely attractive. I'm a photographer. I'd love to take some pictures of you. Are you free some afternoon and we could go to the park?"

b. Photography is a real excuse for stopping a woman, but more than that it gives you a legit way to let her have your phone number (or take hers) so that you can arrange a future meeting for the photo session, or just to discuss the possibility of a photo session.

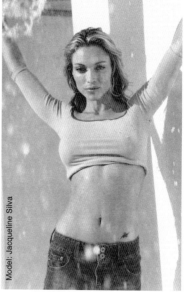

Model: Jacqueline Silva

c. After the photo session you have another meeting assured. She'll be dying to see how the proofs came out, and perhaps she'll want to have a couple enlarged (let her pay for these, unless you're rich) and that means a further get together.

Photographic requirements? You need a good camera. I suggest a 35 mm such as 'Pentax', 'Cannon' or 'Nikon'. You can buy these second-hand at most camera stores. Make sure they are in perfect order, and before you start telling attractive women that you are a great photographer, I suggest you learn to handle the camera, at least competently. A modicum of skill and knowledge is required, but basically any-

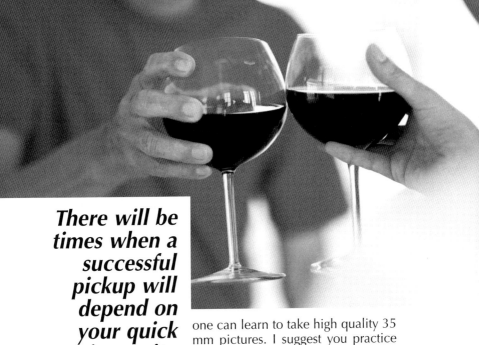

There will be times when a successful pickup will depend on your quick ingenuity.

one can learn to take high quality 35 mm pictures. I suggest you practice on your sister, brother or even the neighbor's dog.

There are of course, thousands of successful pickups made up and down the country, without the use of a camera. I am simply suggesting that taking up photography can aid a man who feels he needs some real excuse for approaching women.

Ever Ready

To be successful at picking up women, you're going to have to practice. Expertise only comes with practice. This means that you are going to have to think picking-up every waking hour. You need to be ever alert, observant and on the prowl.

Remember, that there will be many times when a successful pickup will depend on your quick ingenuity. Once I was having a drink at a local drinking spot when I spotted a beautiful woman at the bar with a tall male escort. I quickly observed that although she was 'with' this fellow she was forever looking around the place at the other customers.

When a new face came in the door, she would turn to see who it was. Clearly, I surmised she was bored to tears with her escort. I all but finished my beer and after

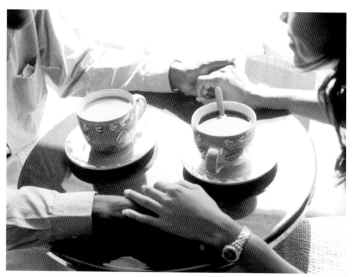

half-an-hour of patience, the fellow left for the washroom. I gulped down the remainder of my drink, hastily made my way to the bar and ordered another beer. "I come in here every night," I said. "You're a new face. Where do you come from?" She managed a warm smile and told me that she was Swedish, and that she was being shown around by a friend.

If you go into a bar, restaurant or coffee house, look around you for pickup opportunities.

She emphasized 'friend' rather than 'boyfriend' so I developed the conversation further and arranged to meet her the following evening. Her friend returned from the washroom no more the wiser, and I vanished from the scene. The next evening the woman and I enjoyed a meal and were together every night of her three-week vacation.

If you walk into a bar, a restaurant or a coffee house, quickly look around you for pickup opportunities. If there are two seats, one next to an old man, and one next to a slender young beauty, then for heaven's sake make the right choice and sit next to the woman. Elementary? Yes, but you'd be surprised at how many fellows will sit elsewhere.

Take (and even make) opportunities. Don't hesitate to follow a woman on an escalator or an elevator. Even if you were originally going to go to another floor, you should get off where she goes. (After all, your chance to strike up conversation exists only as long as you are together or in close proximity. Opportunities can present themselves.) In fact, you could pretend you made a mistake, by cursing your stupidity. Laugh at the situation aloud and contact is made. She'll laugh with you and the pickup is on.

Practice

We have discussed earlier the importance of not appearing too slick and professional when approaching women. This doesn't mean that you shouldn't take every opportunity possible to practice.

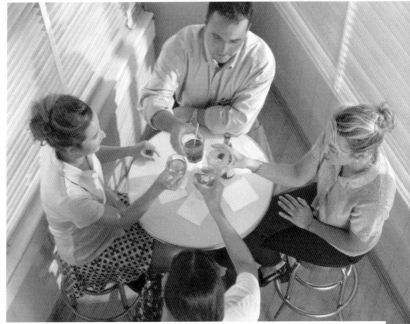

Do not appear too slick and professional when approaching a woman.

If you find yourself sitting next to a woman who is not exactly your cup o' tea, then talk to her any way. I did this once in a Santa Monica pub. The woman was dark haired, short, skinny and not bad looking, but (and I was certain of this) just not my type. I started up a casual conversation. Half-an-hour, and two beers later her girlfriend arrived. She was a bombshell! Blonde, tall, willowy, legs right up to her ass. Naturally, all three of us sat around and enjoyed stories and jokes until closing time. Later on I took the blonde home and arranged to take her out the next night.

Always take advantage of opportunities.

When I picked her up the following evening, she made it clear that she wanted to go to bed. With me! I couldn't believe my luck. And it all came about from my chatting with her girlfriend with whom I had zero interest.

"The girl who shares this apartment with me has gone home to her parents for the weekend," she said. "Let's just stay in and watch TV."

We watched half a movie on the TV and then spent the rest of the night under the sheets.

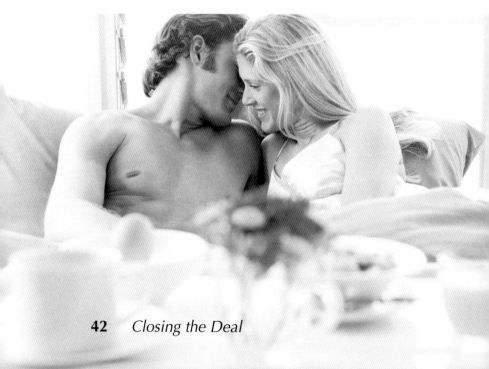

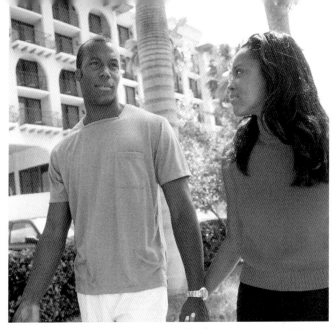

But this story hasn't ended. The interesting thing is that I met the original short, dark, skinny woman again and found that even though she wasn't spectacular looking, that she did in fact have a fantastic personality and a great charm. In getting to know her I found something that was more than skin deep. A new relationship materialized. We actually dated for two years. My advice to you is to always take advantage of opportunities. They often lead to better and bigger things. If you get asked to a party – go. Never turn down a 'gift' of an opportunity to talk to women in a bar, store, library, museum, etc. Talk to everyone, even men! Who knows? They might be waiting for an attractive sister to join them for a drink. And then you're well in!

It has been said that every opportunity taken always leads to two or three more similar opportunities. Don't forget that!

Bottle

(It's English Cockney for courage!)
Have you ever noticed that the thought of doing something daring or dramatic is often worse than actually doing it?

I must have developed the beginnings of a trillion ulcers in worrying about how to approach this or that woman. And yet, when I've actually had the bottle (courage) to go up to a lady and make a play for her favors, it has never been particularly nerve racking.

The thought of 'having a go' has invariably been worse than the approach itself. How, you may ask, does one develop bottle? The answer lies in your action rather than your thinking about the problem. First, you should be prepared for action at all times. Psyche yourself up for pickup opportunities when you go out on the street.

Don't just think about it – get into action!

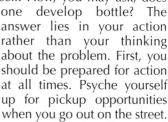

Don't wait until you actually see a pretty girl before you get the adrenalin flowing. As you leave your home, office or car, take note of as many things as you can about your surroundings. Is it a rainy day, cloudless sky, hot, windy, cold? Are there lots of people? Is it rush hour? Any disturbances, accidents, unusual circumstances? Make a note in your mind of how you can relate any of these things to 'lines' that can be used in picking up women.

"Great weather eh?"

OR

"Brr, I wish I had a nice big coat like you ..."

OR

"Did you see that terrible accident down the road, bodies all over the place."

Yes, you will have more 'bottle' if you are prepared, and part of being prepared comes about from feeling confident. If you are the type of person who only feels confident if you have on a jacket and a tie, then for goodness

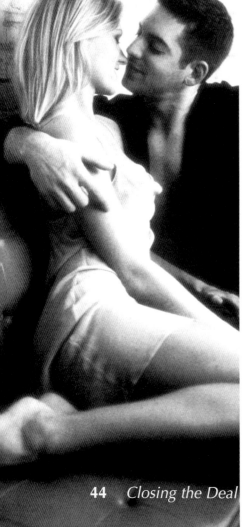

sake wear what you feel best in. Some men only feel confident if they have clean, just-washed hair, or a tanned face. One friend of mine only feels like picking up women if he has been for his regular five-mile run that day. Another only feels confident when he's wearing a white T-shirt and faded jeans. It takes all sorts to make a world.

The thing is that you should do all you can to make your pickup as easy as possible. Don't work under hardships, which with a little effort, you can control. Finally, the thing to remember is: Don't just think about it – get into action. If you feel scared tell yourself that worse things could happen, and that it's not the end of the world, and then without a moment's hesitation do just that. Get into A-C-T-I-O-N!

The thing about 'bottle' is that women love you for it. Even if she is madly in love with someone else, she'll admire you for having the guts to approach her. And rightly so. You, too, should be proud of yourself. For every woman you try to meet, there are literally hundreds of guys wishing they had the 'bottle' to do the same. Women know it takes guts to make a pickup. There have, no doubt, been times when they too have wanted to talk to strange men, but lacked courage to make the first move. Yes, they know you are showing bravery when you stop them 'cold turkey' in the street and they love and admire you for it!

End Piece

The beauty of forever being on the prowl, for women is that you never know what's going to happen next. Honestly, it's amazing. There will of course be failures, but you shouldn't regard them as such.

Women know it takes guts to make a pickup.

Generally, if you are not rude to a woman, she will treat you with courtesy, even though she may not fall for your line. Anyway, she may be getting married the following day. As luck would have it, I once moved in on a fantastic looking woman sitting invitingly alone in a restaurant. As it happened she was quite pleased to talk. But no way was I going to be able to pull her. She was waiting for

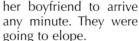

her boyfriend to arrive any minute. They were going to elope.

Another time I was sitting opposite an absolutely perfect creature. She had the most beautiful face I've ever seen and a body that held promises of utter perfect proportion. I was in a dither. My heart was knocking up against my ribs like a caged lion trying to break free. I was going over different lines in my mind but becoming increasingly aware of the fact that I wouldn't be able to spit them out, even if I had the guts to try. My stomach was like jelly.

And then it happened, "You're a Pisces aren't you?" she said. "That's right!" I lied, "How on earth did you know?"

That first chance meeting lead to a hundred days of lovemaking that are etched in my mind forever.

The truth is, of course, that even if you are devastatingly handsome you are not going to be picked up everywhere you go. Even in this liberated age it is still the woman who has to be approached. But unexpected things do happen, and when they do, you'll jump in the air with sheer ecstasy.

One friend of mine was following an exquisite brunette along a crowded walkway. She had a head of rich black hair and perfect olive skin, with the biggest brown eyes you've ever seen. With each step her bottom seemed to coax his lust to near boiling point. She crossed the road and he followed in hot pursuit. But somehow she managed to weave between the traffic and he got caught in the middle of the road. In the short time he took his eyes off her to check the oncoming cars and buses, she was out of sight. Lost. My friend searched the neighboring stores and even asked the porter of a local block of apartments if she had been in. All to no avail. It seemed that he would never see her again.

Depressed and fed up he decided to drown his sorrows with a drink at a nearby wine bar, and who should be serving behind the counter but this same sexy girl. "Christ!" he exclaimed with unembarrassed surprise. "So this is where you got to!" He went on to tell her that he had seen her just a short time before and explained how suddenly she had disappeared. "Now!" he joked. "Now, that I've found you I'm never gonna let ya go!" She smiled affectionately and they've lived together happily ever since.

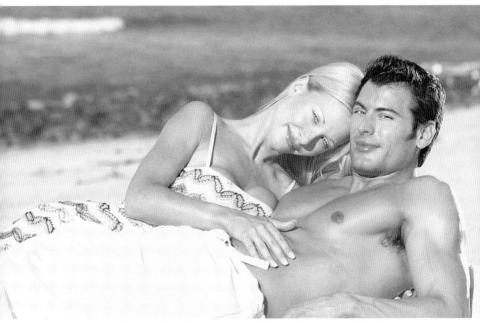

Don't be afraid to talk a beautiful woman. You just might be her 'White Knight.'

<u>Contributing photographers</u>
Alex Ardenti, Robert Kennedy,
David Paul, Rick Schaff, Rob Sims